7-Day

Detox Challenge

7-Day Detox Challenge

7-Day
DETOX
CHALLENGE

Detox Your Body In 7 Days

CHALLENGE SELF

http://www.ChallengeSelf.com

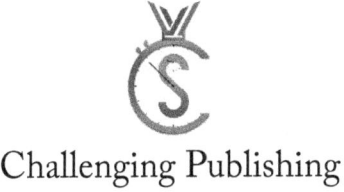

Challenging Publishing

ISBN 978-1-535-45642-5

Printed in the United States of America

First Edition

YOUR OVERVIEW:

7-Day Detox Challenge

Your Instructions:

How to Best Approach This

This book is not meant to be read entirely in one sitting, but for over the span of each day.

Why? The reasons are relatively simple. We do want you to benefit from the information, which will take time to process, and we do not want to overwhelm you with all the applications of what you will learn. At the same time, we don't want to make this another breezy one-time read, and then you're off to do something else, forgetting your new knowledge without ever applying it to anything.

Now you probably will be eager and tempted to go through this all in one sitting, but we're encouraging you to take it slow. Remember that the best way to approach this is <u>one day</u> at a time. Do not move on to the next day until you have completed its previous day(s).

This approach is effective because if you truly want to improve, you need to remain grounded in the process. There is no such thing as a magic pill; there is continuous conditioned improvement. Rome wasn't built in a day. Likewise, none of the top performers, best athletes, and successful people in the world have gotten to where they are in a day. Breaking things up into separate days supports an ongoing process and builds upon each previous day's progress to bring it all home in the end.

Of course, each individual's experience will be different. You may or may not accomplish your goal after the entire trial is over. In that case, you can repeat it all again starting from Day 1 to the last day.

If you commit yourself, you will see improvement. Are you ready to proceed on to your challenges? Then let's begin!

P.S. If you ever need to contact us, you can always reach out to us at our official website:

http://www.ChallengeSelf.com

7-Day Detox Challenge

<u>Your Challenge:</u>

Remove Toxins

A lot of people might look at detoxing as a waste of time. Heck, why not just go on a diet or make yourself start eating healthier?

If you think that, you do have a point—eating healthier *does* make things easier in the long run. But you can't ignore the fact that permanently adopting healthier eating habits just isn't easy and most of the time people end up failing at it.

With a detox plan, you're doing the same thing a healthy diet does, only faster.

It shouldn't take a genius to decipher the meaning behind the word "*detox*."

- "de-" and "tox" together means getting rid of toxins and impurities that have built up in your system. Some of these toxins are disease-causing *even if you only have them in low concentrations.*

In other words, detoxing is not something people do just for fun—there are very good reasons behind it.

There are even signs you may notice that tell you when you *need* a full-body detox.

Specialists, such as Dr. Sara Gottfried, MD, consider the following symptoms to be among those you want to watch out for: bad breath, congested sinuses, fluid retention, cravings, increased belly (or bloated feeling), moodiness, fatigue, itchy skin, insomnia, and even depression.

Need any more persuasion? Here's a list of benefits you can get from your detox:

–Regain your vitality and energy. By following a detox plan, you'll feel relieved, lighter, and more enthusiastic about the things you love to do.

–Improve your mood. With fewer toxins in your system, your health and mood will be improved before you know it.

–Lose weight. This plan focuses on cutting a lot of bad habits and keeping you on a very specific (healthy!) eating regimen, so you may even lose a few pounds as an unexpected bonus!

–Rejuvenate your skin. The detox dedicates an entire day of the plan to teaching you how to care for your abused skin, as well as incorporating several other skin-care exercises throughout the week.

Detoxifying your body is one of the best things you can do for it. The detox plan is simple to set up, doesn't need any surgeries or medical bills, and **you can actually feel it working** (during the colon detox, for instance).

So go ahead proceed on and you'll be all set to start your detox!

Before you begin your detox plan, there are certain things you need to know:

1.) **A detox plan is only effective if you eat the right foods during the entire program.** You'll want to focus especially on catabolic foods, as they'll help your body burn calories faster (many of the fruits and vegetable mentioned here and later are high-grade catabolic foods). To help you in your selection, the following fruits and vegetables should be included in your detox shopping list:

–Foods high in sulfur (helps remove toxins effectively): Brussels sprouts and garlic (fresh bulb garlic).

–Foods high in glutathione (a protein that helps detoxify the liver): carrots, tomatoes, grapefruit, spinach, walnuts, and avocados.

–Natural diuretics: asparagus. Eat this vegetable—preferably raw—to combat bloated feelings.

2.) You need to be aware that <u>there is a possibility that you might feel some discomfort or other side effects during the detox</u>. Edward Group, DC, NP, DACBN, DCBCN, DABPN, identifies the following side affects you might experience during the early stages of the detox plan, particularly during the colon detox phase:

–Vomiting, nausea, dizziness/dehydration, bowel perforation, infection, mineral imbalance, or headache. **If you notice any of these symptoms, stop the process immediately and seek treatment.**

3.) It's important that you use filtered water instead of tap. Dr. Gottfried recommends that you filter your water before drinking it anyway, as the Environment Working Group has found about 316 different chemicals in tap water (mainly chemicals used to disinfect it), and you don't want any of them in your body—*detox*, remember!

4.) You'll also need to cut coffee, alcohol, cigarettes, and sodas for the same reason. On the same note, Alejandro Junger, MD, recommends replacing red meat with white meat (organic chicken and turkey, for instance), since it's slightly easier for your digestive system to handle.

You are now ready to start your detox! Get ready to cleanse your body of all the processed foods (and the results of unhealthy lifestyle choices) that are slowly killing your system. Just remember, pretty much all you need is the right food, clean water, and, of course, a good helping of self-discipline.

As a disclaimer: We recommend that you consult your doctor prior to attempting any type of detox plan. Detoxifying your body is a rapid change and a major lifestyle shift, and the consequences of these changes can sometimes lead to discomfort or hospitalization.

It is not our intention to encourage you to start a detox plan if you suffer from a life-threatening or chronic disease.

Seeking professional advice first is always recommended.

7-Day Detox Challenge

DAY 1:

The Colon Detox

Colon Hydrotherapy

With our modern "processed" diet, it's become almost impossible for our bodies to evacuate food effectively. To put it bluntly, as a whole, we're way more constipated and bloated than our grandparents. You can see it when you look at old photos: people back then were so much thinner and better-looking, weren't they?

It doesn't seem fair, does it? Well, with a little work, you can make a step in the right direction by giving your system a boost with a good <u>colon detox</u>.

You may ask, *why start with the colon?*

According to David Williams, DC, also a medical researcher and biochemist, all detox plans should begin with the colon. This is because, in order for your liver, intestines, and the rest of your system to be cleansed, your colon and intestines have to be free from any "leftovers" (fecal matter) still in your intestines. When you evacuate the fecal matter still in your colon, you're getting rid of undigested waste and promoting better nutrient absorption.

There are several types of colon detoxes, such as the colon hydrotherapy—performed by a qualified hydrotherapist—a colema, which you can perform at home, and several oral cleanses.

The most advocated form of the detox, however, is the **colema**. Specialist Bernard Jensen, DC, Ph.D., recommends it as the gentlest and most effective form of cleansing.

However, if you're not comfortable doing a colema, other options are discussed here, too.

Despite which cleanse you use, though, **the best time to start the detox is going to be during the weekend,** in the morning or early afternoon. This way you'll have enough time not only to make sure you're comfortable with the process (to make sure there are no side effects) but also to rest and proceed with the last phase of the process without having to rush.

The Colema Method

If you're going for a colema, <u>you'll need to start early by taking an intestinal cleanser</u>—1 scoop diluted in apple juice and taken as per the instructions—<u>for a week before the</u>

<u>detox</u>. This will loosen your stool and ensure that the cleanse can be fully effective. There are several other items you'll need, though, as well as a slightly different variation you might consider.

What you'll need:

–You'll need a colema cleansing kit, which comprises a board, a 5-gallon bucket, rubber hoses and a colema tip, a pillow, soft pads, and a blanket (for comfort).

–Warm (body-temperature), filtered water (remember, no tap water). This is the simplest solution you can use.

Another variation on the cleanse will need:

–Garlic water. (This is ideal for people who suspect the presence of parasites in the colon. One indication of this is rectal itching.) For the specified

5 gallons of water, you'll need 6 to 10 cloves of minced garlic. (Make sure the garlic is thoroughly liquefied before mixing it into your water—you don't want your colema tip getting clogged up.)

Performing the Colema:

Fill a gallon bucket with body-temperature, filtered water. Place the bucket on a sturdy surface, about 4 feet above your colema board (which should be on the floor). Siphon your warm water through the tube. It should be flowing without a problem through the rectal tip. Use organic olive oil to lubricate the tip, then position yourself on the board and start inserting the tip into your rectum (make sure you insert no more than 3 inches of it). When it's in place, start massaging your belly so the liquid can do its work through the colon. Try to hold the liquid in as long as possible, but when you feel you can't hold it in any longer, evacuate it into the toilet. You'll probably notice a lot of waste (fecal matter) during the first round.

Restart the process. Again, hold it in as long as you can, then evacuate. Repeat the procedure until you've used the whole 5 gallons—the entire thing should last between 45 to 60 minutes.

If you wish to see what comes out of your system, you can opt not to flush the toilet right away; it's up to you—maybe it'll be a wake-up call.

*Important Note: Unless you're already highly experienced, you should either have the colema performed under the supervision of a medical-trained professional or have it done for you, especially if it's your first time.

Oral Method 1: Colon-Detox Capsules

Again though, if you're unable to do the colema, or you just aren't comfortable with it, there *are* **oral cleanses** you can try instead.

Colon-detox Capsules: The first oral option is simple. All you have to do is take a pill. That's it! You'll need to go to the pharmacy and speak to a pharmacist for advice on the best and safest pill, but then all you have to do is read the instructions on the label—consult a physician if you have any further questions—and take the pill as recommended in the instructions.

*Be advised that most of these products contain licorice, which can lead to high blood pressure. If you notice any discomfort after using oral colon-detox pills for the first time, stop the process and consult a doctor immediately.

Oral Method 2: Natural Alternative

If you're leery of taking pills, or just want a more natural alternative, you can also use a diet cleanse. All you'll need for this one is water and assorted vegetables and cereals (grains, not Cheerios). No lie; it's that easy. The water gives you the liquid and lubrication your body needs in order to flush toxins and waste, and the raw vegetables contain the enzymes necessary to keep you regular. The same applies to fiber-rich foods, which also help soften your stool and encourage the body to expel waste. (It's important, though, that you use all natural, organic foods. Trying to detox is pointless if you're putting in more toxins and chemicals at the same time.)

What you'll need:

- 2 cups broccoli

- 1 cup spinach

- 2 cups diced carrots

- 1/2 cup non-GM corn

- 1 cup kale

- 2 cups purified water

Use a grinder to mix all your raw vegetables, then add the water and mix again. That's all there is to it!

You'll also need 10 to 12 glasses of water (purified) and a good selection of fiber-rich foods to eat throughout the day. (You can overdo it on water, however, so be careful with such a big intake. Nausea, headaches, and muscle spasms or cramps can all be symptoms that you've "overdosed.")

You'll be sipping on your raw vegetable "smoothie" and eating your fibers at intervals throughout the day, so by about midday you should start feeling the need to use the restroom.

Organize your menu by this schedule: 4 glasses of your veggie smoothie during the day, interspersed with 10 to 12 glasses of water and 3 separate meals of your "fiber-food" of choice.

Aftercare and Maintenance

- After you've completed the **colema**, you'll need to do a sesame-oil insert to maintain the health of the mucosal layer in your colon. (You can use a disposable enema bottle.)

You'll need to lie down on your side, on the floor, and squirt the oil into your rectum (squeeze the bottle so that all the oil comes out). When you've done that, roll to the left side first, then lie flat on your back so the liquid is distributed evenly. 3 to 5 minutes should be enough time for the oil to be absorbed into your colon. (Try to resist passing gas so that the oil can be absorbed appropriately.) If, after 5 minutes, you feel liquid still trying to come out, simply evacuate it into the toilet.

Clean your kit in the shower with water and alcohol and let it dry in the bathtub.

- With the **detox capsules** it's important to make sure you drink lots of water afterward. You should still be eating plenty but nothing too heavy. Avoid foods like bread, cheese, chips, meat, or anything fried. The best foods are going to be ones you can easily digest and evacuate—soup, for instance.

You're also going to want to avoid *doing* anything heavy today. Just let yourself rest, and give your body time to "re-stock" with good bacteria.

- With the **natural cleanse** the instructions are pretty much the same. Try to avoid heavy foods, (try noodles or non-spicy soups, yogurt, apple sauce, etc.), drink lots of water, and make sure you spend plenty of time resting up.

7-Day Detox Challenge

DAY 2:

The Liver Detox

Phase Two

Now that you've finished the cleanse specifically for the colon, you can move on to the next step of the program—also known as the liver detox.

The colon came before so every impurity flushed out of your liver can be properly evacuated from your system, without the risk of being released into the bloodstream (which can happen if you have fecal matter left inside your colon).

Since it's a full-body detox, **the colema/oral method can only be done on the first day**, as it affects the healthy bacteria that promote proper colon and intestinal functioning. Doing it otherwise might disrupt the next cleanses on your schedule. The liver detox requires energy and a stable digestive system, so it's best to get the colon cleanse out of the way first.

Now that you've got that fun info down, you can get on to the liver cleanse. Again, there are numerous ways to detox your liver. Your options include a detoxifying herbal supplement, the "lemonade diet," a liver or gallbladder flush, and, last but not least, the liver-detox diet.

Unfortunately, several of these techniques can have very uncomfortable side effects, such as nausea, vomiting, and even surgery. So, to make things simple, Edward F. Group, DC, NP, DACBN, DCBCN, DABPN, recommends the liver-detox diet, which focuses on certain fruits and vegetables that specifically contribute to liver cleansing.

***Note**: The liver has to process all of these toxins you're flushing from your body during the detox. If your system is weak, or you've been on an unhealthy diet for a while, your liver may be unable to handle the sudden stress. The best way to prevent this is to give yourself a healthy diet to follow for some time prior to attempting the cleanse.

The Liver Smoothie

A "liver smoothie" sounds pretty odd, doesn't it? In reality, though, since there are quite a few fruits and vegetables included in the list for the aforementioned diet for detoxing your liver—and since you'd have to work *really* hard to eat all of them in one day—we've simplified the diet into an all-inclusive smoothie recipe. Put all the ingredients into a blender and you're good to go!

What you'll need:

- 3 quartered beets (aids the liver in processing toxins)

- 3 chopped carrots (also aids the liver)

- 2 cups leafy greens of your choice (keeps heavy metals and toxins from accumulating)

- 1 cup dandelion greens (increases the production and flow of bile)

- 1 quartered organic lemon (helps the body transform and expel toxic material)

- 1 cored and sliced apple (helps cleanse and release toxins from the digestive tract)

- 1 cup chopped purple cabbage (aids in enzyme production in the liver)

- Filtered water (2 to 3 cups)

- 2 tablespoons coconut oil (forms an ideal source of healthy fat when detoxing your liver)

Other foods recommended are: grapefruits, artichokes, walnuts, garlic, and olive oil (to name a few). Garlic and olive oil would definitely make a strange addition to your smoothie, but if you're feeling adventurous, why not give one of these extra ingredients a try?

Prepare your smoothie: When you add the ingredients to your blender, start with the largest chunks of fruits and veggies (the quartered beets and apples), then add the rest—including your coconut oil. Add water until the pitcher is about 3/4 full, then blend on high until the whole mixture is liquefied. When you're happy with the consistency, go ahead and drink the smoothie immediately in order to take full advantage of its nutritional benefits.

This one smoothie should be plenty for the day, but, for maximum effectiveness, you'll want to drink it before you start your daily activities.

Follow-Up Diet

It would be a waste not to reinforce your liver-detox smoothie with a healthy diet, so to follow it up, plan the rest of today's meals according to this list:

–Foods that are loaded with potassium, such as bananas, tomatoes, avocadoes, and Swiss chard. Potassium is good for maintaining liver processes, fighting heart diseases and depression, and promoting good water balance.

–Foods that are rich in vitamins B-6, C, D, magnesium, and iron. Try a boiled sweet potato for lunch; they're high in these nutrients, and, when boiled, the sugars they contain are released into the bloodstream through the liver and won't cause a spike in your blood sugar.

–Real beef liver is also good, as it's high in quality protein, iron, B vitamins (good for bones, vision, brain health, and energy), and antioxidants (good for fighting inflammations).

There are no known side effects to the liver smoothie, but for today you *will* want to stick with the foods listed above and avoid any processed foods, as they'll put a lot of strain on your newly cleansed liver. You're supposed to be supporting it, remember, not re-loading it with junk food.

And don't forget to supplement these recommended foods with plenty of protein and healthy fats—you're not done yet, and you'll need to have plenty of energy and strength in order to handle the rest of the program.

7-Day Detox Challenge

DAY 3:

The Lymphatic Detox

Below the Surface

If you're living a typical modern, unhealthy life, your skin is going to be one of the major casualties. When you smoke, drink more than your fair share of "adult beverages," and don't get to bed until 1:00 every night, you're going to have skin breakouts, acne, blemishes, premature skin aging, and dark circles under your eyes.

Noticed any of that? Well, this is when a lymphatic detox comes in handy.

But what exactly is a lymphatic detox? So far it sounds like a skin detox, right? Since it involves both the skin surface *and* the membranes and organs underneath, however, it's technically a lymphatic detox.

But don't worry, there *is* a detox specifically for the skin that comes in later.

For now, though, internationally recognized leader in natural health, John Douillard, DC, CAP, who specializes in both Ayurveda (a traditional Hindu system of medicine) and sports medicine, claims that the lymphatic detox starts with your digestive detox, so Day 3—right after the colon and liver detoxes—is the perfect time to focus on it.

Today you're going to make sure those toxins you worked on flushing during the two previous days are also eliminated through your lymph.

Deep Surface Cleansing

To set you up for the lymph detoxification, have your liver detox smoothie in the morning (the same ingredients you used yesterday), and make sure you drink lots of water during the day.

Instead of sticking to your "liver diet," though, today you're mostly going to be working on cutting out all foods with colorings, sugar replacements, preservatives, and other additives. In other words, in your meals today you're going to have to **religiously avoid sodas, fast foods, coffee, and anything else that might fall under the "junk food" heading**. Instead, be prepared to replace them with any or all of the foods from the following list:

–**Citrus:** Fruits such as tangerines, oranges, and grapefruits possess powerful enzymes and are high in vitamin C, which supports the body and promotes digestion. Today you'll either need to eat 3 servings of these fruits or combine them into a citrus-fruit salad—

you can even smother it with honey, if you like—and snack on it during the day.

–**Berries:** Cranberries, strawberries, and blueberries, for instance, are rich in detoxifying benefits and help keep your skin hydrated.

–**Greens:** (You can reduce them into a green smoothie for extra benefits.) Most green veggies help protect your body from harmful chemicals and toxins on a daily basis. They also contain vitamins A, C, and K, magnesium, iron, and protein.

–**Herbs and spices:** Spices such as turmeric, ginger, cinnamon, coriander, and black pepper all contain antioxidants. It's a double bonus—you can spice up your meal and give your health a boost at the same time.

–**Chia, hemp, and flax:** These seeds all contain antioxidants and are also a good source of Omega 3—a fatty acid excellent for lymph flow.

To make it simple, you'll also need to avoid red meat, alcohol, coffee, and starchy foods, as they're harder for your body to process. Instead, substitute two or three of the foods listed above.

Manual Surface Cleansing

As well as eating carefully, you're going to have some manual work to do for this cleanse.

Exercise and perspiration are both excellent for the lymph (and for helping it eliminate toxins), so make sure you get in at least a short, brisk walk or some other light exercise that gets your heart going and your sweat flowing.

Before you shut down for the night, you'll also need to do some dry skin brushing in order to further stimulate your lymphatic system, exfoliate your skin, increase your circulation, improve your digestion, and even work as a stress-reliever.

Using a brush with stiff bristles and a long handle (so you can reach the hard-to-get areas on your back), gently brush your skin, starting from your feet and working your way up. (When brushing, make sure you always brush toward your heart, and avoid spots such as your face and genital area.) At the end of the session—it should last about 20 minutes—your skin should have a healthy pink color (not red). If you start looking like a lobster after the first few brushes, you're doing it too hard.

Make sure you do this 3 to 4 hours before your bedtime, as the process will leave you energized and might make it hard to sleep. And you need your sleep if you want a healthy glow the next morning.

To finish up the detox, drink a large glass of water.

*Note: You may find yourself feeling a bit dizzy, what with all the flushing and brushing you've been doing. If you notice this, try eating a bowl of fruit and honey, then resting for a while. If the feeling persists, stop the detox and wait for another time.

If you don't get the dizzy feeling, or you manage to get rid of it, then you can move on to the next step.

DAY 4:

The Kidney Detox

Flush It!

Today you'll be working on a <u>kidney detox</u>.

As you probably know, your kidneys are highly important organs that help rid your body of toxins found in the blood. When kidneys stop functioning normally, calcium inside them can start to build, eventually turning into kidney stones. There's no need to tell you how painful this is (you probably get the idea).

In order to prevent it, then, a frequent kidney detox is a huge step.

You don't have to worry about making the liver-detox drink today—this step of the cleanse has its own slate of special liquids that will replace the previous smoothies. What you *can* do, though, is have a dry brushing session first thing in the morning, and make sure to eat something that includes tomato paste (chicken breasts in tomato sauce, for instance) for lunch or dinner. (Remember, tomatos are high in potassium.)

But these are just side issues. Your main goal today will be to focus on drinking your kidney-detox liquids and adding kidney-promoting foods to your meals.

Clean the Filters

To start you off, your first detox drink will be the watermelon flush.

What you'll need:

- 6 cups fresh watermelon, including the rind and seeds

The preparation is pretty simple: reduce 6 cups of fresh watermelon to juice, grinding in the rind and seeds. (You'll be sipping on this all day, so make sure your serving sizes are small enough to cover 2 glasses in the morning, 2 in the afternoon, and 1 at night.)

For the remainder of the detox, you'll need to drink lots of water—filtered, of course—and stick to these guidelines:

- Eat lots of berries (for their antioxidants and antibacterial benefits).

- Add barley to your meals. It's rich in fiber, magnesium, and manganese; it helps you stay regular and lowers the cholesterol in your blood.

- Avoid red meat, alcoholic beverages, and any beverages containing caffeine.

Expand Your Options

Some nutritionists, such as Edward Group (remember him?), also recommend adding other kidney-detox drinks to your list—cranberry, beet, and lemon juices, for instance, which, when drunk regularly, all help fight the formation of kidney stones.

In other words, if you get tired of watermelon . . . on top of watermelon . . . on top of watermelon, you can alternate with cranberry, beet, or lemon juice (whichever you prefer). You'll have to be careful that the cranberry juice is 100% natural (with no additives), but the lemon juice you can make yourself with real lemon, pure water, and, of course, without sugar. Beet juice may be harder to find, but it will also work well.

The kidney detox sounds pretty simple, right? Well, that's because it is. And if this sounds good, then you'll be relieved to know that the next steps of the full-body detox are also relatively simple.

7-Day Detox Challenge

<u>DAY 5</u>:

The Lung Detox

Human Ventilation

You've gone through the colon, liver, and kidney detoxes, and now you're going to move on up to the lungs. Your lungs perform an average (for adults) of *20,000 breaths a day!* Needless to say, you want them to stay in good working order.

Luckily for that goal, the guidelines for the <u>lung detox</u> are pretty basic:

- Aerate your space. Keep your windows open when you're in a room and breathe slowly and deeply, completely filling your lungs with air.

- Practice deep breathing. Lie on your back in a calm place and slowly breath in (counting to 5), then breath back out (counting to 5 again). Repeat this process 8 times per session, and make sure you get in at least 3 separate sessions a day.

- Stick to the diet options outlined below, including the beverages you'll be using for this detox. (What, you haven't come to expect it yet?) According to the American Lung Association, healthy foods are a necessity if you want to have healthy lungs and healthy breathing. Duh, right? But you'd be surprised how many people don't take this into account.

So, with these guidelines, you can go ahead and get started on the detox.

Internal Air Purifier

The first step is to prepare a beverage to combat lung inflammations.

- For this you're going to use licorice tea. To prepare it, add a teaspoon of licorice powder to 1 cup of hot water. Cover your glass, steep for 10 minutes, then drink.

This tea fights lung inflammation, but once you've had that, you'll want to put together another vegetable "smoothie," this time to help rejuvenate your lungs.

What you'll need:

- 1 handful of watercress (look for it in the salad section of the grocery store)

- 1 turnip

- 1 lemon

- 2-3 carrots

- 1 cup of clean water

Combine these ingredients the same way you put together your other smoothies, then enjoy. (You'll only drink it once today, so adjust your portions accordingly.) These particular vegetables combine to make the perfect detox drink for soothing swollen breathing passages and promoting lung health.

For the Rest of the Day

Since you're not going to survive all day on these beverages, however, here are your other food options for today, put together in a simple menu:

- Have a bowl of organic bran cereal for breakfast—along with your rejuvenating smoothie—and top it with blueberries (a strong anti-inflammatory).

- Fix yourself some variety of fish for lunch or dinner, along with a broccoli and spinach salad (omega-3 and greens).

- Have a helping of grapes with the remaining meal, and remember to keep sipping on your licorice tea (have 2 cups for the day).

To end the detox on a good note, take a 25-minute walk—at a normal speed—making sure to take deep, full breaths of fresh air. The main reason people get out of breath is that they don't use their lungs properly. This walk, and the other breathing exercises included above, should help you get your lungs working to their full capacity before you move on with the detox.

Before bed tonight, sip on another cup of warm licorice tea (not too soon before bed, though—you don't want to be in the bathroom all night).

*Note 1: Licorice is not suitable for you if you are pregnant, diabetic, have high blood pressure, or suffer from any type of kidney disease. Use ginger tea instead (unless you are taking medication for high blood pressure).

- To prepare the ginger tea, you'll need hot water and fresh, grated ginger. Steep the ginger for 10 minutes, then enjoy.

*Note 2: If you're a smoker, you'll need to avoid the cigarettes during the entire process, preferably from the very first day of the detox plan, if not before.

7-Day Detox Challenge

7-Day Detox Challenge

DAY 6:

The Skin Detox

Save Your Skin

That's right, we've come back to the skin detox. Your skin is what's holding your body together, remember, and as such . . . well, it's pretty important.

The lymphatic detox before focused on what's directly *under* the skin, but the skin itself needs work too. You've been flushing out toxins all week and most of it has been eliminated through your urinary tract or colon, but what about your pores?

Your pores are also outlets for your body, and when they get clogged with toxins and other materials, you can be exposed to acne and other skin breakouts. You helped it a little when you worked on getting up a sweat during the lymph detox, but given the huge variety of things that can harm your skin—pollution, for example—it's important to include it in the detox.

The skin detox has no specific beverages you'll need to take (besides water), so you're going to move back to the kidney-detox smoothie in the morning in order to both continue the kidney detox for maximum effectiveness and balance with the liver detox. Since you've had liver detox smoothies more than once since day 2, you'll want to make sure you take an equal amount of the kidney smoothie during the week—preferably in the morning—so that everything's balanced.

Once you've had your smoothie, you can start your skin detox. Your schedule today will consist of cleansing the skin and, wait for it . . . following with the appropriate diet.

Skin Care

So, besides a bar of soap, how *do* you cleanse your skin?

- To answer that question, skin-care specialists, such as Dennis Gross, MD, recommend starting with clay (in the morning). Clay removes the sebum that your skin naturally produces—and which can build up and clog your pores—as well as the dehydrating residue your skin collects from using tap water. After the clay, you'll want to apply an organic moisturizer—one that contains both sunscreen and antioxidants. Dr. Gross also recommends applying a serum containing chelator (helps keep your skin tone and texture clean) before you add the moisturizer.

There are also quite a few foods that are helpful during the skin detox:

- Water is one of the most important because of its ability to prevent constipation and bloating, which cause puffiness and paleness of the skin. To get the full benefits, make sure you drink around 10 glasses of water at intervals throughout the day. (Again, be sure not to overdo it.)

- Fruits and vegetables containing carotenoid pigments—carrots, tomatoes, oranges, squash, etc.—are especially good for the skin and should always be part of the skin detox. Dark, leafy greens (rich in antioxidants) are also beneficial.

- Finally, extra virgin olive oil (raw), and other foods rich in omega 3 (and low in omega 6—they're both necessary, but generally you have more omega 6 than you need) help maintain your hair and skin and should be included as often as possible.

So, for your meals today, start with a couple (at least) of fresh tomatoes and carrots. To make the veggies on your list more palatable, try putting them together as the mother of all salads. You should also try using olive oil on your salad and adding some roasted salmon to your dinner menu.

To top off the cleanse, finish up with another glass of water.

7-Day Detox Challenge

DAY 7:

The Final Purge

The Big Day!

You've made it to Day 7! Feels like you need some confetti and cheering, doesn't it? But remember, you're not quite done yet. Today you're going to put the separate detoxes together (most of them), and end with a big detox elimination before bed.

You've learned a lot over the past week and worked through a lot of detoxes, but since this is only a 7-day plan, you'll have to repeat some of the most important processes to guarantee results. (Detox plans such as the liver, kidney, and lymphatic detoxes, for instance, are continued over several days during the week.) So today, you'll organize your cleanse according to this schedule:

- Start with your dry skin brushing. Repeat the procedure you learned on Day 3—remember to brush gently—starting with your feet and brushing toward your heart. Brush for about 20 minutes, then move on.

- Have yourself a liver smoothie. This will be your first smoothie of the day. If you still have room when you're done, you can go ahead and eat breakfast (make sure it's healthy and all-natural).

- Sip on some licorice (or ginger) tea before lunchtime. This is for your lung detox, so make sure you also remember to air out your space and practice your deep breathing.

- Have a kidney smoothie—or one of the recommended juices—along with a light lunch of organic kidney cooked in tomato sauce, and boiled sweet potatoes. This way you get a combination of the liver and the kidney cleanse.

- Drink a glass of water and snack on some baby carrots or cocktail tomatoes. Remember, all of these promote skin health.

- Fix a healthy dinner, and have a citrus salad— oranges, grapefruits, and tangerines—as a dessert.

- To finish up with the skin cleanse, take a good shower and make sure to wash your hair thoroughly. (This is really only best if you have a water filter on your showerhead. Tap water contains chemicals, remember.)

- After the 7 days specified in this detox program, continue the lymphatic, liver, and kidney detox plans for another 2 days. As we said earlier, these plans normally go on for days. (If you want to keep it organized, make sure you stick with the liver smoothie in the morning and the kidney smoothie in the evening.)

Once you've worked through these steps, you'll be officially finished with the detox!

Continuing Your Detoxes

You've officially finished your cleanse, but there are several things you should bring away from this experience:

1.) For maximum health, you should consider cleansing your colon at most once every 2 months. **This is not something that should be done all the time, as it can be harmful to the bacteria in your digestive system.**

2.) **Enrich your daily diet** with more vegetables, fruits, and foods containing omega 3, such as salmon.

3.) **Remember to exfoliate twice a week.** Sunblock should be applied during hot seasons, and products with a chelator can (and should) be used daily to promote a healthy glow. Drink plenty of water during the day and try to avoid alcohol and smoking.

4.) **Learn to detox regularly,** even if you already live a relatively healthy life. You can't protect yourself from everything, so there are still plenty of ways your body can accumulate toxins.

Doctors and nutritionists, such as Vilma Brunhuber, MD, recommend detoxifying your body many times during the year and for long periods of time. Some of the detoxes—such as the colon and liver detoxes—are often recommended to last as much as 2 weeks or more!

Longer *is* generally better, but since this might seem too excessive to keep up, we've put together this detox plan to simplify things for you. The 7-day detox should be repeated approximately once every 3 months. This is because the lymphatic cleanse should be used every new season (about every 3 months), and the colon benefits best from being cleansed every 2-3 months. And with these cleanses, you're going to get the best results if the other cleanses are there to supplement them.

Above, if you recall, we recommended continuing the detox for a few more days, but, in the future, you can go ahead and stick to the original 7 days. Since this was probably your first detox, we added the extra time in order to make sure you get the maximum benefits and effectiveness.

7-Day Detox Challenge

7-Day Detox Challenge

<u>Challenge Complete:</u>

Body Renewed

Our bodies do a great job of getting rid of toxins every day—it's part of the natural process.

Unfortunately, with our unhealthy modern lifestyle, **we tend to over-abuse them,** weakening them or causing them to shut down completely.

This is where a detox plan can be a life-saver.

Think of your body like your car. Every 3,000 miles or so, your car needs an oil change and a good going-over, right?

Well, *your body is the same way*. A head-to-toe detox gives your over-worked systems a lube job, cleansing them thoroughly and getting them back into good working order.

If they're going to continue keeping you healthy, they need maintenance every once in a while—just like your car.

Waiting until you come down with kidney stones or liver failure shouldn't be an option. If you want optimum health, you should give your body a detox at least every 2 months.

Remember, it's not just about the inside. True beauty (or good looks, for you guys out there) starts with health, and you can give yourself a boost in the right direction with a periodical detox.

Get healthy today with your detox!

7-Day Detox Challenge

7-Day Detox Challenge

<u>Your Feedback:</u>

Was Your Challenge Accomplished?

Congratulations on completing all your challenges! You should be proud of yourself for making it this far. For that, give yourself a big pat on the back! :)

Now, we have a huge favor that we would like to ask you. We want to know: have you accomplished the goal you established when you began this trial?

No two people are the same, so results will always vary.

If you have seen the results you wanted, give yourself another pat on the back, and please kindly share your testimonial wherever you purchased this book. If you let us know about it, we have a small free gift to offer you as a token of our appreciation.

However, if you aren't satisfied in any way, we urge you to please contact us directly to let us know what could have been different to help you achieve better results. We want to know if there is any way we can further help you.

Plus we are very easy to get a hold of online!

Official Website:
http://www.ChallengeSelf.com

Social Media:
https://www.facebook.com/ChallengeSelf
https://twitter.com/MyChallengeSelf
https://plus.google.com/+Challengeself

"YOU" are our main priority, and we're all here for you!

Take care! And always challenge yourself!

www.ingramcontent.com/pod-product-compliance
Lightning Source LLC
Chambersburg PA
CBHW060640290526
45793CB00001B/336